D1077562

What you really need to know about

BREAST CANCER

Dr Robert Buckman

with Tereza Whittaker

Introduced by John Cleese

A QUANTUM BOOK

This edition published by Silverdale Books,
an imprint of Bookmart Ltd,
Blaby Road, Wigston, Leicester, LE18 4SE

Copyright © 2000 Marshall Editions Developments Ltd

This edition printed 2006

This book is produced by
Quantum Publishing Ltd.
6 Blundell Street
London N7 9BH

ISBN 1-84573-124-7

QUM1344

Printed in Singapore by
Star Standard Industries Pte Ltd

Cover photography: front GJ Images/ The Image Bank; back GJ
Images/ The Image Bank

The consultant for this book, Dr Clare Vernon MB Chir MA
FRCR, is a consultant in clinical oncology working at Imperial
College School of Medicine and the Hammersmith Hospital,
London. She qualified from Cambridge and St Bartholomew's and
her main research interests centre on patients with breast cancer.

The information and recommendations contained in this book are intended to
complement, not substitute for, the advice of your own GP. Before starting any
medical treatment, exercise programme or diet, consult your GP. Information is given
without any guarantees on the part of the author and publisher, and they cannot be
held responsible for the contents of this book.

Contents

Foreword   4
Introduction   6

Chapter 1: Symptoms & Causes
What is breast cancer?   10
Causes of breast cancer   14
Types of breast cancer   18
Breast cancer research   22

Chapter 2: Diagnosis
Assessment and diagnosis   26

Chapter 3: Treatment & Care
What influences treatment?   34
The holistic approach   36
Principles of treatment   38
Surgical treatment   40
Reconstructive surgery   48
Adjuvant treatment   50
Systemic therapy   54

Chapter 4: Living with Cancer
Looking and feeling good   64
After treatment   68
Regular checks   70
Talking to children   72
Palliative care   74

Understanding the jargon   76
Useful addresses   78
Index, Acknowledgements   79

Foreword

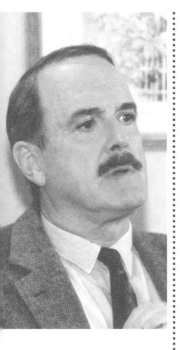

Most of you know me best as someone who makes people laugh.

But for 30 years I've also been involved with communicating information. And one particular area in which communication often breaks down is the doctor/patient relationship. We have all come across doctors who fail to communicate clearly, using complex medical terms when a simple explanation would do, and dismiss us with a "come back in a month if you still feel unwell". Fortunately I met Dr Robert Buckman.

Rob is one of North America's leading experts on cancer, but far more importantly he is a doctor who believes that hiding behind medical jargon is unhelpful and unprofessional. He wants his patients to understand what is wrong with them, and spends many hours with them—and their families and close friends—making sure they understand everything. Together we created a series of videos, with the jargon-free title *Videos for Patients*. Their success has prompted us to write books that explore medical conditions in the same clear, simple terms.

This book is one of a series that will tell you all you need to know about your condition. It assumes nothing. If you have a helpful, honest, communicative doctor, you will find here the extra information that he or she simply may not have time to tell you. If you are less fortunate, this book will help to give you a much clearer picture of your situation.

More importantly—and this was a major factor in the success of the videos—you can access the information here again and again. Turn back, read over, until you really know what your doctor's diagnosis means. In addition, because in the middle of a consultation you may not think of everything you would like to ask your doctor, you can also use the book to help you formulate the questions you would like to discuss with him or her.

John Cleese

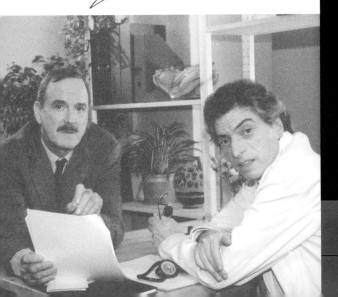

Introduction

DOs AND DON'Ts

✔ Find out as much as you can about the subject so you can make an informed choice about your treatment.

✗ Don't be afraid to ask questions and seek help.

Breast cancer is the most common cancer in women, affecting one in 10 women at some time in their lives. The likelihood of developing it becomes greater as you get older, and it is most likely of all to develop in women who have passed the menopause.

Information and support

As with most cancers, the earlier breast cancer is detected and diagnosed, the better the chances of successful treatment. One of the best ways of ensuring that breast cancer is spotted as early as possible is by being breast aware—check your breasts once a month so that you become familiar with their usual appearance, contour and feel, and so better able to seek early medical advice if there are any changes in either breast that are out of the ordinary. This book also gives you information about other symptoms and signs that could indicate breast cancer and so prompt you to see your doctor at an early stage in the disease.

The most serious problem with breast cancer is that it may spread to distant parts of the body. Doctors are not able to predict precisely whether a particular breast cancer will spread, but there are certain features that indicate whether the chance of spread is high or low. On the pages that follow you will read about the different types of breast cancer, how doctors estimate the chance of spread and the various treatments you may be offered.

Exploring treatment options

For most women, the first treatment is surgery to remove the lump in their breast. The treatment given after this very much depends on the chance of spread. You may be offered radiotherapy, chemotherapy or hormone therapy, or a combination of treatments. This book tells you why each treatment may be offered, its beneficial effects and also the possible side effects you may experience. Armed with this knowledge you can make an informed choice about your treatment—if you know that your cancer has a high chance of spreading and a particular treatment can reduce that chance, you may be more likely to accept it if your doctor recommends it. Whereas if the chance of spread is low, and therefore the chance that you have already been cured by surgery is high, you may be less motivated to accept more treatment. It is always your choice.

A normal life

Remaining as well as you can will be one of your prime concerns after breast cancer. You will be given exercises to help you regain mobility in your arm and shoulder after surgery, and you should not be afraid to ask for any help you may need to deal with the anxiety and depression that can occur after cancer treatment. Looking good is important too. An attractive wig and a good prosthesis— if you need them—can do wonders for your self-esteem and help you get on with this new phase of your life.

BREAST CANCER CARE

This charity offers information and support to all those affected by breast cancer or who have breast health concerns. It runs a telephone helpline and has a website full of practical advice and news on the latest research. Details can be found on page 78.

Chapter

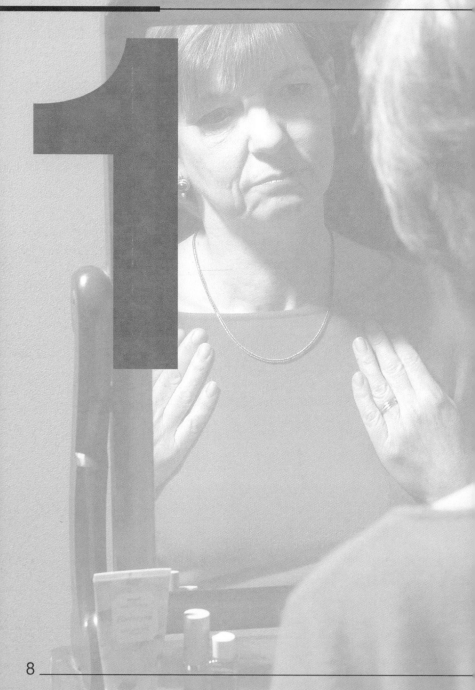

SYMPTOMS &
CAUSES

What is breast cancer?   10

Causes of breast cancer   14

Types of breast cancer   18

Breast cancer research   22

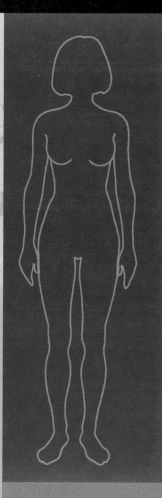

What is breast cancer?

✓ Breast cancer is not a single disease, it is a group of conditions, which include a number of different types of cancer.

✓ Some breast cancers grow quickly and spread through the body. Others grow more slowly and remain in one place.

A cancer is a group of abnormal cells growing together in an uncontrolled way, invading and damaging healthy tissues. A group of growing cancer cells form a lump, which is called a tumour. If the tumour is in the breast it is called breast cancer.

Cells are the body's building blocks—all our organs and tissues are made up of many different types of cell. The body keeps itself healthy through cell growth and renewal, and almost all cells need to be replaced at regular intervals. Normal, healthy cells grow, divide and die under the control of genes. If there is a change (mutation) in any of the growth-controlling genes, a healthy cell turns into an unhealthy, tumour cell. These changes make the cell look abnormal when it is looked at under a microscope. As well as changing shape, the cells behave differently. They grow uncontrollably, and divide to form more and more tumour cells.

Tumours can be benign or malignant. Benign tumours grow slowly, do not spread to other parts of the body and are not life-threatening. Malignant tumours are harmful. They grow more rapidly, and the cells may spread to other parts of the body where they form secondary tumours (also known as metastatic tumours).

The structure of the breast

The breasts are made up of glandular tissue held together by connective tissue and fat. The glandular tissue consists of lobules and ducts. During breast feeding, the lobules fill with milk which then flows along the ducts leading to the nipple. The ducts and lobules are supported by the connective tissue. Breasts change through a woman's life. Young women have more glandular tissue than older women, making their breasts firmer. As women get older, the proportion of fat in their breasts increases and the breasts tend to droop more.

The breasts sit on top of the chest muscles, outside the ribcage. The arteries carry oxygen-rich blood to the breasts, while the veins drain the blood away. This draining of blood through the veins sometimes provides a route for breast cancer to spread through the body.

The lymphatic system

The breast also has a lymphatic system, which plays an important role in filtering harmful substances. It consists of lymph nodes (the main ones are in the neck, armpits and groin) linked by vessels that contain a fluid called lymph. Lymph flows around the body in these vessels in the same way that blood flows in the veins and arteries.

UNDER THE SKIN

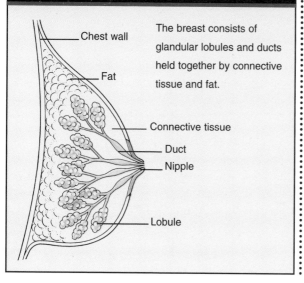

The breast consists of glandular lobules and ducts held together by connective tissue and fat.

Chest wall

Fat

Connective tissue

Duct

Nipple

Lobule

What is breast cancer?

✓ Screening refers to tests done to look for cancer. These include breast examination and special X-rays called mammograms.

✓ Remission is when the cancer has responded to treatment and is under control. It is not the same as cure, but if the cancer stays away for more than 10 years it may be considered cured.

Women and cancer

One in three people in the world will develop some form of cancer during their lifetime, and in women, this cancer is most likely to be cancer of the breast. More than 25 percent of cancers (one in four) diagnosed in women are breast cancer. Lung cancer, ovarian cancer, and cancer of the colon or large intestine are the next most common cancers affecting women.

Is breast cancer on the increase?

In the UK, approximately one in 10 women of all ages will develop breast cancer at some time in her life, and about 30,000 new cases are diagnosed each year. Many people are worried that breast cancer is becoming more widespread, because a few years ago the figure quoted was one in 12 women. The disease is, in fact, becoming

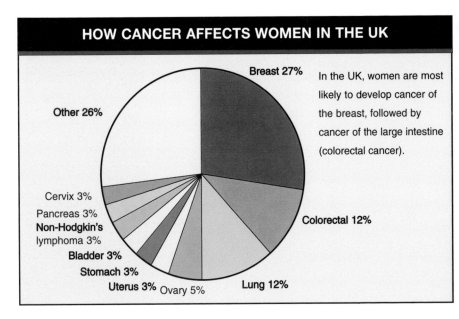

HOW CANCER AFFECTS WOMEN IN THE UK

Breast 27%

Other 26%

Cervix 3%
Pancreas 3%
Non-Hodgkin's lymphoma 3%
Bladder 3%
Stomach 3%
Uterus 3% Ovary 5% Lung 12%

Colorectal 12%

In the UK, women are most likely to develop cancer of the breast, followed by cancer of the large intestine (colorectal cancer).

a little more common, but some of this increase may be explained by the success of screening programmes in diagnosing breast cancer at a much earlier stage than was previously possible. It is not entirely clear why the rate of breast cancer is so high in the UK, but we do know that the Western lifestyle plays a role (see p. 14).

Who gets breast cancer?

The overwhelming majority of breast cancers occur in women—over 99 percent. The next most important risk factor is a woman's age. The disease is found more frequently in older women. At the age of 25, the risk of developing breast cancer is approximately one in 20,000. By 35, this has increased to one in about 600 and at age 50 the risk is one in 50.

Older women who have passed the menopause are the most likely of all to get breast cancer. This is why breast cancer screening programmes are aimed at older women. The national breast screening programme in the UK monitors women between the ages of 50 and 64, offering routine mammograms (see p. 28) every three years. Screening programmes such as this aim to pick up the disease as early as possible, before the tumour has had time to grow and spread. The sooner a tumour is found and cancer is diagnosed, the better the chances of treating it successfully.

What is the outlook?

Although breast cancer can be a life-threatening disease, if it is detected early enough, when the cancer is still small and before it has had a chance to spread to other parts of the body, up to 80 percent of women will be treated successfully and cured.

YOU REALLY NEED TO KNOW

◆ Breast cancer is the most common form of cancer to affect women.

◆ The risk of developing breast cancer increases with age and it is most common in post-menopausal women.

◆ If breast cancer is detected early, there is a good chance that it can be cured.

What is breast cancer?

Causes of breast cancer

No one knows for certain what causes breast cancer. We do know that the disease is much more common in countries where people have a Western lifestyle than it is in developing countries. However, we do not know precisely what it is about the lifestyle in these countries that causes women to develop breast cancer. There is some evidence to suggest that it is partly due to diet—particularly to the higher proportion of fat in the food we eat—but more research needs to be done.

Even though we do not know exactly how breast cancer is caused, we do know some of the things—the risk factors—that make a particular woman more liable than the average woman in her country to develop breast cancer. Being exposed to a risk increases your chances of developing cancer, but not everybody in a high-risk group will automatically do so.

Increasing age

Age alone does not cause cancer, but the incidence of breast cancer increases the older you get. Eighty percent of breast cancers occur in women over 50. It may be that initial damage to cells took place many years previously, and that the cancer took time to develop.

Age at first pregnancy

If you have your first child before the age of about 18, you have a lower chance of developing breast cancer. We do not know why this is, and it does not necessarily mean that early pregnancy is a good idea. Having a child at such a young age can have serious consequences of its own, for example on the mother's education and employment prospects. The protection against breast cancer is only partial—it is a weak protector rather than

INCIDENCE OF BREAST CANCER

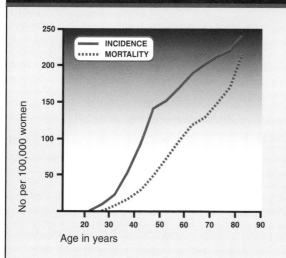

Age is the most important risk factor for developing breast cancer and incidence increases dramatically with age.

a total preventer. So no woman should have her first child in her teens simply because she wants to prevent breast cancer developing.

Number of menstrual cycles

The total number of menstrual cycles you have in your life is related to your risk of getting breast cancer, because it affects your exposure to oestrogen. If your periods start when you are young and your menopause occurs late, the overall number of years of exposure to oestrogen is higher than for women who have a later first period and earlier menopause. This is known to increase the risk of developing breast cancer.

1

**YOU REALLY
NEED TO KNOW**

◆ No one knows for certain what causes breast cancer.

◆ A number of risk factors are known to increase your chance of developing breast cancer—but do not inevitably lead to your developing the condition. Some of these factors are beyond your control.

Causes of breast cancer

Causes of breast cancer

Breast feeding

Women of all ages who breast feed their babies gain a small amount of protection against breast cancer. But breast feeding is only a weak protector, and some research suggests that even this is not noticeable unless breast feeding has continued for several years.

A previous breast lump

Lumps in the breast are very common. Most non-cancerous lumps in younger women are caused by benign tumours called fibroadenomas. In older women, non-cancerous breast lumps are more likely to be caused by cysts.

Neither fibroadenomas nor cysts normally pose any risk to health and do not increase the chance of getting cancer later. However, if a benign breast lump shows certain changes, called atypical hyperplasia (see p. 19), when looked at under a microscope, there seems to be a slight increase in the chance that the woman will later develop breast cancer, even though that particular lump has been removed. Experts believe that atypical hyperplasia is a sign that the cells in the breast are generally unstable, so there is a greater than average chance that later on another part of the breast (or part of the other breast) will develop a cancer.

Can the pill cause breast cancer?

The available evidence suggests that the contraceptive pill probably does not contribute to the development of breast cancer, and certainly not if you take it for less than 10 years. What matters is the dose of oestrogen in the tablet, and modern pills contain much lower doses than earlier pills. Although there may be a small increase in risk with long-term use, the benefits of the pill, which include protection against ovarian cancer, still definitely outweigh the risks.

Prolonged use of any oestrogen therapy, including hormone replacement therapy (HRT), taken to protect against the effects of the menopause, may increase the risk of breast cancer very slightly. In the past, HRT contained high doses of oestrogen, but modern versions use much smaller doses, and there does not seem to be any increased risk of breast cancer in the first 10 years of use. Oestrogen also protects against heart disease and osteoporosis, which may pose a much greater threat to life and health than any increased risk of breast cancer.

RUNNING IN THE FAMILY

◆ A woman with a first-degree relative (mother or sister) who had breast cancer is twice as likely to develop the disease compared with someone with no family history of breast cancer. If that relative suffered from breast cancer at a young age, i.e. before the menopause, the relative risk is greater. Women whose aunts or grandmothers had breast cancer also have an increased risk, but to a lesser extent.

◆ The breast cancer genes BRCA1 and BRCA2 (probably present in fewer than one in 20 women) indicate that a woman has about an 80 percent chance of developing breast cancer and a 50 percent chance of passing the gene on to her daughters. Gene testing is not routinely available, but it might be worthwhile to test women in families with a high incidence of breast cancer to check for either of these genes.

YOU REALLY NEED TO KNOW

◆ Taking the contraceptive pill for less than 10 years does not increase the risk of developing breast cancer.

◆ Using HRT or another form of oestrogen therapy might increase the risk of developing breast cancer, but it does offer protection against heart disease and osteoporosis.

Causes of breast cancer

Types of breast cancer

When you are discussing your symptoms with your doctor, ask him to write down the names of any medical words or expressions you do not recognize or understand.

If after studying your doctor's notes you still don't understand everything, ask for a further appointment.

Cancer of the breast can be classified in many different ways, depending on what the cells look like under a microscope. Not all of the visible differences affect the way the cancer behaves and so do not influence the choice of treatment, but one feature is of great importance—whether the cancer is invasive or not.

Invasive disease

Breast cancer begins inside either one of the ducts of the breast or one of the lobules. With invasive cancer, the pathologist (who studies the cells under the microscope) can see the cancer going through the wall of the duct or through the lobule out into the surrounding breast tissue. So "invasive breast cancer" means cancer that is spreading out of the duct or out of the lobule. Most breast cancers are of the invasive type.

Non-invasive disease

Some cancers stay inside the ducts or lobules. These are called "in situ" (Latin for "in the original position"). In situ cancers behave differently from the more common invasive cancers, and may not cause any further trouble once they have been removed. They are also treated differently from the invasive types of breast cancer.

Ductal carcinoma in situ (DCIS) can grow as a small lump in just one place, or it can develop in more than one duct or part of a duct. Lobular carcinoma in situ (LCIS) is cancer growing inside one of the lobules. Although an in situ cancer tends not to become invasive itself, if a woman does develop one it means there is an increased risk of her developing another cancer elsewhere in the breast in the future, so she will be regularly monitored.

Premalignant disease

Normal cells grow, divide and die in a regular way. Sometimes an overgrowth of normal-looking cells form a lump called hyperplasia. Although this condition is harmless, it can lead to atypical hyperplasia, where the cells lose their normal shape and appearance. Atypical hyperplasia is also usually benign, but some types may be premalignant—a warning sign that cancer may develop.

Other types of breast cancer

Other, rarer types of breast cancer include Paget's disease, where a slow-growing cancer produces changes in the nipple; cystic carcinoma, which is a cancer growing within a cyst; and inflammatory cancer of the breast, which causes redness, swelling and pain. It spreads quickly and often there is no evident lump.

◆ Non-invasive cancer is called "Carcinoma in situ". This type of cancer is limited to a duct or lobule.

◆ "Invasive carcinoma" is cancer that has spread into the surrounding breast tissue and can spread to other parts of the body.

◆ There are two main types of invasive breast cancer. The most common begins in the cells lining the ducts and is called "invasive ductal carcinoma". Invasive cancer arising from the lobules is called "invasive lobular carcinoma".

TYPES AND SITES OF BREAST CANCER

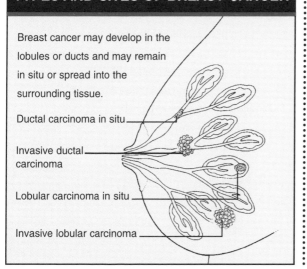

Breast cancer may develop in the lobules or ducts and may remain in situ or spread into the surrounding tissue.

Ductal carcinoma in situ

Invasive ductal carcinoma

Lobular carcinoma in situ

Invasive lobular carcinoma

Types of breast cancer

Types of breast cancer

How breast cancer spreads

If an invasive cancer has spread from the duct or lobe where it began into the surrounding breast tissue, this is called "local spread". Local spread may take place over many years, or more quickly. As the number of cancer cells increases they form a lump (tumour). The tumour keeps growing and at some point will be big enough to be felt in the breast tissue. The size of the tumour when it is first detected is important when deciding on treatment.

In slightly less than two-thirds of cases, breast cancer does not spread beyond the breast and in many cases may be cured by surgery (with or without radiotherapy).

WHERE SECONDARY TUMOURS ARE FOUND

Breast cancer probably spreads through the body in the bloodstream. If it does, secondary tumours (metastases) develop. These are usually in the bones, the spinal cord, lungs, liver, ovaries or brain. For a few women, symptoms from the secondary tumour, such as bone pain, are the first indicators of their breast cancer.

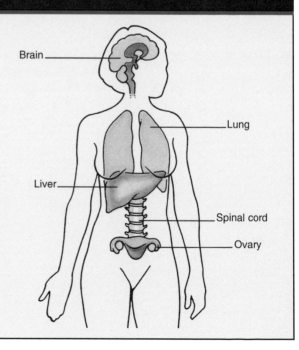

Brain

Lung

Liver

Spinal cord

Ovary

How secondary tumours develop

With any type of cancer, the first lump that forms is called the primary tumour. In breast cancer, most primary tumours are found in the upper, outer part of the breast. From here, the cancer may spread to form tumours in more distant parts of the body. These are called secondary tumours (or metastases).

Cancer is probably spread by the bloodstream, although we are not yet certain exactly how. We do know that the lymph nodes in the armpit act as signals (or markers) as to how likely a particular breast cancer is to spread. This is why you should examine your armpits as well as your breasts during breast self-examination (see p. 27) to try and detect any nodes that may have become involved. Affected lymph nodes become swollen and enlarged.

If the lymph nodes are not involved, the chance of the cancer spreading is relatively low. If the lymph nodes are affected, the chance of spread is higher, although the cancer almost certainly does not spread from the lymph nodes themselves.

Where does it spread to?

Once cancer cells have spread from the breast to other sites in the body, they start to grow, forming the secondary tumours. If it does spread, breast cancer most commonly spreads to bones, the liver or a lung, and sometimes to other places such as the ovaries, the spinal cord or the brain.

It is because of the possibility of spread that cancer treatment often includes chemotherapy (see p. 54). Chemotherapy is used to try and destroy all cancer cells in the whole body, not just those in the breast.

(see p. 27) · (see p. 54)

YOU REALLY NEED TO KNOW

◆ Local spread is when the tumour spreads into the surrounding healthy breast tissue.

◆ Distant spread to other parts of the body is called metastasis. Breast cancer cells may spread to the bones, lungs, liver, ovaries, spinal cord or brain. The tumours that grow at these sites are called secondary tumours or metastases.

Types of breast cancer

Breast cancer research

✓ It can make you anxious to be told that there are different ways of treating your breast cancer. Make sure you have all the information you need.

✓ You may be invited to join a clinical trial. These trials are scientifically designed to try and find out more facts about a disease so that new treatments can be developed. You do not have to take part, but you may choose to if you know what the purpose of the trial is.

Nowadays, it is relatively easy to diagnose breast cancer, but once the diagnosis is made things become less clear cut. There has been a lot of research on the subject, but it has not yet provided all the answers and there are still many things we do not know about breast cancer.

Research into the causes

One of the most important discoveries in breast cancer research was finding two breast cancer genes in 1994 (see p. 17). Women in families who carry these genes have an increased tendency to develop breast cancer. Further research is needed to find out exactly how these genes work and experts hope this will lead to a breakthrough in understanding and possibly preventing

COPING WITH THE DIAGNOSIS

◆ The diagnosis of breast cancer can cause feelings of shock, disbelief, fear and anxiety. You are entitled to a second opinion, and you are likely to be referred to a specialist breast unit. If you are not, insist that you are.

◆ Once the diagnosis has been confirmed, finding out more about your disease will help you to make the right decisions. Take time to find out as much information as you need to help you make informed choices.

◆ You may be feeling anxious when you see the doctor, which will not help you to ask the right questions or remember what you are told. Write your questions down beforehand and take notes of the answers or bring a tape recorder with you.

breast cancer altogether. At least 90 percent of breast cancers, however, are not caused by these genes and we still do not know exactly why the disease develops.

Research into the types

To predict how a cancer will behave and so decide on the best course of treatment, we need to know as much as possible about its nature. New tests to identify the exact type of cancer are currently being developed. These include looking at the cancer's sensitivity to hormones and measuring other markers that indicate how aggressive (likely to spread) it is.

Genetic markers (oncogenes) that appear to influence growth rate, and therefore outlook, have been found in some breast cancers. The most common is ERB-B2 (see p. 60). New therapies act directly on proteins produced by these oncogenes to interfere with the cancer's growth.

Research into the treatment

Because breast cancer includes a range of conditions, there are a number of treatment options (see p. 38). Doctors now try to save the breast by offering smaller operations and using other treatments in addition to surgery. There is still debate about the best combinations of treatment to use and when to use which treatment, so you may find that your treatment differs from that of someone else you know.

What you can do

Every woman has the right to decide how much she wants to know about her illness and to choose between the different treatments offered to her. Informing yourself of all the facts allows you to choose what is best for you.

(see p. 60)

(see p. 38)

YOU REALLY NEED TO KNOW

◆ The tests used to diagnose breast cancer are reliable and are available to all women in the developed world.

◆ Breast cancer patients also need help in dealing with the emotional impact of the diagnosis.

◆ Do not be rushed into making decisions about treatment. Take what time you need to make the right choice for you.

Breast cancer research

Chapter

2

DIAGNOSIS

Assessment and diagnosis   26

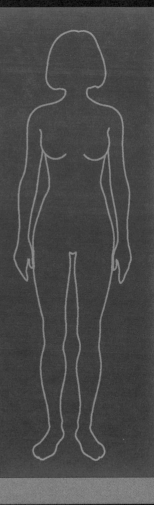

Assessment and diagnosis

✓ Benign cysts in the breast are more likely to cause discomfort or pain than a cancer is.

✓ In a very rare form of cancer, inflammatory breast cancer, the whole breast suddenly becomes red and feels hot and swollen.

The way most women (or their partners) find a cancer in the breast is through feeling a lump. For many women the lump has not caused any symptoms and seems to have appeared quite suddenly. Lumps in the breast are very common, and nine out of 10 are not cancer. But because of the risk of cancer, if you find a lump—with or without symptoms—you should see your doctor promptly (within a few days).

Most breast cancers do not cause any specific symptoms, so it is difficult for a woman to reliably distinguish a benign lump from a cancer. But there are a few symptoms that may suggest breast cancer.

Nipple symptoms

If a tumour grows near the nipple it may make the nipple become inverted (drawn inwards). If one or both of your nipples has been inverted since puberty and you can evert them (pull them outwards), there is no need to worry. It is only when one nipple becomes inverted later in life and cannot be easily everted that there is reason to suspect cancer.

Occasionally breast cancer may cause bleeding from the nipple, or a rust-coloured or bloodstained discharge. Most bleeding or discharge is caused by benign conditions, such as cysts. Even so, if you notice a discharge, have it checked by your doctor.

Skin symptoms

Sometimes you may notice that skin over the lump seems to be attached to the lump when you move your arm. This is called tethering. Accumulation of fluid in the tissues of the skin may make the skin look pitted, rather like the peel of an orange.

BREAST SELF-EXAMINATION

Regular breast self-examination helps you become familiar with your body so you will be able to spot any changes.

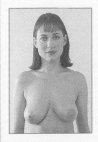

1. Undress to the waist and stand in front of a mirror (left). With your arms loosely by your sides, look for any alteration in the shape, size and symmetry of your breasts and nipples.

2. Raise your arms above your head and again check for changes. Turn sideways to see your breasts in profile (right).

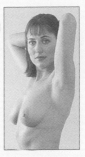

3. Now put your hands on your hips and push downwards, so that your chest muscles tense up. Look again for any of the signs listed above.

4. The next part of BSE is better done lying down. With one arm behind your head, use the flat of your fingers to feel firmly for any lump or thickening.

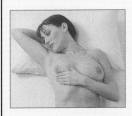

5. Work your way around in a spiral, covering all areas of the breast (left). Remember also to check your armpits. It is important that your doctor follows the same steps if you attend the surgery for a check-up. If you are not happy with the way your doctor examines you, ask for a second opinion, or bring it up for discussion.

YOU REALLY NEED TO KNOW

◆ Some women naturally have lumpier breasts than others. Breast self-examination makes you familiar with what is normal for you.

◆ Any change in your breast, nipple or armpit needs to be examined by a doctor.

◆ Breast self-examination is best done once a month, at the end of your period, when the breasts are softer.

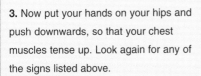

Assessment and diagnosis

Assessment and diagnosis

Mammography

When an X-ray of the breast is taken to be used to look for cancer, the process is called mammography. The X-ray is called a mammogram. A mammogram can pick up very small tumours before they have spread into the surrounding breast tissue and lymph nodes, even before they can be felt as a lump.

In the UK, the national breast screening programme offers routine mammograms to women between 50 and 64 years every three years; women over 64 can request them. The programme aims to pick up as many cancers as possible as early as possible. Younger women have denser breasts, which do not show up as well on a mammogram, so only those who have a high risk of breast cancer are offered regular mammograms.

WHAT DOES A MAMMOGRAM SHOW?

A mammogram is a picture of the breast on X-ray film. Cancer shows up as a white lump, a group of little white specks, or a combination of the two. The results are not always absolutely clear—the radiologist may have difficulty interpreting the mammogram, or there may be an area that does not show up well. If this is the case, you may be asked to come back for another mammogram.

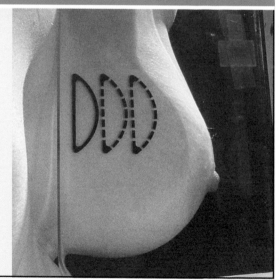

How is a mammogram done?

The nurse will ask you to undress to the waist, and wipe your breasts clean of any talcum powder or deodorant. The radiographer will then press each breast in turn between the X-ray plate and the compressor plate for a few seconds and take an X-ray. Your breasts need to be as flat as possible for a good-quality picture. Mammography must be done by an expert, and should only be carried out at a specialist unit.

Many women find mammography uncomfortable and a few even find the process quite painful, but it helps if you are prepared and know what to expect in advance. Occasionally, your breasts may feel bruised for a few days afterwards.

Ultrasound scan

An ultrasound scan is a picture created using sound waves instead of X-rays. It is not used routinely in screening for breast cancer because it is not as good at detecting cancer as a mammogram. However, it may be used as an extra test in some cases, to get as much information as possible about abnormalities seen on a mammogram. Ultrasound is good at picking up cysts, so it can be helpful for younger women (under 35) who have a lump that is most likely to be a cyst.

Magnetic resonance imaging (MRI)

Magnetic resonance imaging builds up a computerized picture from the way the body's tissues bounce back magnetic waves. Researchers are currently looking at how MRI may best be used to detect breast cancer. It may also be able to tell us about the type of cancer and help predict its behaviour.

2

YOU REALLY NEED TO KNOW

◆ If you are over 50, you should have a mammogram at least every three years.

◆ Most breast cancers show up on a mammogram, even very early in the disease.

◆ Ultrasound is not used as a screening test for breast cancer because fewer than half of all breast cancers can be seen on the scan.

Assessment and diagnosis

Assessment and diagnosis

Fine needle aspiration cytology takes a sample of individual cells and cannot show if a tumour is invasive or in situ.

A biopsy sample contains a group of cells joined together, so it is possible to tell whether the cancer cells have spread from the lobule or duct into the surrounding tissue.

At specialist breast clinics fine needle aspiration cytology and biopsy can be done on the same day.

Cytology

All suspicious breast lumps found during a mammogram must be examined more closely. A pathologist looks at cells from the lump under a microscope (this is called cytology) to see whether or not they are malignant. Cancer cells look different from normal cells.

Fine needle aspiration cytology

In fine needle aspiration cytology (FNAC), cells are withdrawn using a thin needle. With very small lumps, the specialist may use ultrasound or an X-ray to make sure the needle is in the right place. FNAC can show whether an area is a solid lump or a cyst—if it is a cyst, fluid will be drawn off and the cyst will collapse. Fluid from a cyst can be sent for analysis to make sure that there are no cancer cells in it.

Aspiration is usually done without anaesthetic, so you will feel the needle going in. As with most injections, the skin is the most sensitive part, and the aspiration itself is not painful. Asking questions and discussing your fears can help to make the procedure less stressful. There may be some internal bleeding and your breast may feel tender and bruised for a few days. The bruising may be enough to show up on X-ray, so mammograms are always done before fine needle aspiration.

An aspiration takes only a few minutes. You may get the results the same day, or you may have to come back. If the result shows abnormal cells, the next step is a biopsy.

Biopsy

In needle biopsy (also called a core biopsy or a tru-cut biopsy), a piece of tissue about 2.5 cm long and the diameter of a pencil lead is removed under local anaesthetic, using a thicker needle than the one used for FNAC. If the suspicious area is small, the biopsy may be done under X-ray guidance to make sure the right area is sampled. The pathologist then cuts the tissue into thin slices and examines them under the microscope. It is a bigger, slightly more invasive procedure than FNAC. Applying pressure or ice to the site once the needle has been removed will help to reduce bruising.

If there is any doubt about the diagnosis after mammography, FNAC and core biopsy, an open biopsy may prove helpful. This is a larger version of needle biopsy, done in hospital under general anaesthetic. If the whole lump and some surrounding tissue is removed, this is called an excision biopsy or lumpectomy.

FINE NEEDLE ASPIRATION

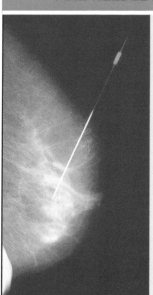

After cleaning the skin, the specialist (usually the breast surgeon) holds the lump firmly and inserts a fine needle into it, rather like giving an injection. He or she then sucks up (aspirates) some of the cells into a syringe before taking the needle out and smearing the cells on to a slide. The cells are then examined under a microscope.

YOU REALLY NEED TO KNOW

◆ Cells taken from a breast lump are examined under a microscope. Cancer cells look different from normal cells.

◆ Fine needle aspiration and biopsy are always done by experienced professionals.

◆ Fine needle aspiration and needle biopsy may be uncomfortable and cause some bruising and internal bleeding, but they are not usually painful.

Assessment and diagnosis

Chapter

3

TREATMENT & CARE

What influences treatment?   34

The holistic approach   36

Principles of treatment   38

Surgical treatment   40

Reconstructive surgery   48

Adjuvant treatment   50

Systemic therapy   54

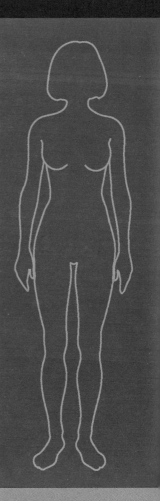

What influences treatment?

✓ Different cancers respond in different ways, so some treatments are more effective than others.

✓ Tests and investigations help the doctor to choose the most effective treatment.

Each type of breast cancer behaves in a different manner. But there are two crucial questions in deciding which treatment is best in each particular case. First, is the chance of distant spread (spread to other parts of the body) high or low? And second, what can be done to reduce that chance?

How doctors predict spread

The chance of distant spread will influence your doctor's recommendations and your choice of treatment options. If your cancer has a high chance of spreading to other parts of your body, and if a particular treatment can reduce that chance, your doctor will recommed that treatment more strongly—and you may be more likely to accept this recommendation. If the chance of spread is low, you may be less motivated to accept a particular treatment.

PREDICTING THE CHANCE OF SPREAD

These factors all help to predict the chance that breast cancer will spread:

◆ Whether the tumour has spread to the lymph nodes in the armpit, and if so how many are involved

◆ The size of the original tumour. This refers to the size as measured when it has been removed—the apparent size before the operation may be misleading

◆ Laboratory tests on the tumour for hormone receptors. These tests are not always done, particularly if the original tumour was very small

◆ Other tests, including tests on the blood, that are done in some cases

3

Doctors cannot tell every woman with breast cancer whether her particular cancer will spread or not, but they can give some estimate as to whether the chance of spread is high or low. Three features are routinely used to help in that prediction: whether the cancer has spread to the lymph nodes in the armpit, and if so how many of them are affected; the size of the tumour; and whether the tumour is receptive to hormone receptor tests.

Tests you may be offered include a chest X-ray, a blood test, to see if the liver is involved, and a bone scan to show any "hot spots" where tumour cells may be growing. Other possible options include tests to show how many cells are actually multiplying at the time and any invasion into the lymph vessels. A blood test may also be done to measure substances called CEA, CA 15-3, CA 19-9 and others, as rising levels may indicate that the cancer is recurring or spreading.

Can the outcome be predicted?

It is very difficult to say with certainty what the outcome of a particular treatment will be for a particular individual. For example, comparing figures from two studies may suggest that one form of treatment has a higher survival rate after five years than the other. But the first study may have involved far fewer women and, if repeated on a larger scale, would prove to have a much lower survival rate. Because of this uncertainty, you should try not to rely on information from an impersonal source, such as TV, newspapers or magazines. You need to get your information from someone who can explain what any statistics mean in your case and can talk through your treatment options with you, answering any questions you may have.

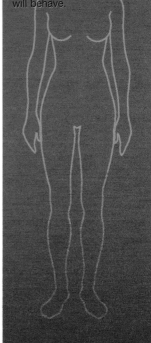

YOU REALLY NEED TO KNOW

◆ The earlier breast cancer is diagnosed, the better the chances of successful treatment.

◆ It is impossible to predict exactly how an individual cancer will behave.

What influences treatment?

The holistic approach

Medical staff are now aware of the need to consider the person as a whole, rather than just deal with her disease. The team looks at the emotional, social, spiritual and financial aspects of treatment as well as the physical.

All patients are entitled to the best possible treatment. For women with breast cancer, this starts with diagnosis. If there is a possibility that you have breast

THE BREAST CANCER TEAM

You will be treated by a team of professionals, including some or all of the following:

GENERAL PRACTITIONER (GP)
Usually arranges the first referral to a specialist breast clinic.

ONCOLOGIST
A cancer specialist, who advises on overall treatment. A clinical oncologist is trained in giving radiotherapy and chemotherapy, a medical oncologist gives chemotherapy only.

RADIOLOGIST
A doctor specializing in the study of X-rays and other imaging techniques. He or she will interpret your mammogram.

PATHOLOGIST
A doctor specializing in the effect of disease on body tissues, and how cells look under the microscope.

RADIOGRAPHER
Trained to use X-ray machines. Some also give radiotherapy.

cancer, your doctor needs to arrange a timely referral to a specialist centre. At the larger breast cancer units, you may get a confirmed diagnosis in one day. Even when you need to wait for a firm diagnosis, there is no need to make any decisions about treatment until you know for sure what your diagnosis is. In most cases up to three weeks delay in starting treatment will not alter its effectiveness.

BREAST SURGEON

A specialist in breast surgery. Usually does the fine needle aspiration and biopsy. Some do reconstructive surgery.

BREAST-CARE NURSE

Nurse with special training in dealing with breast disease. Can tell you what to expect and give support and advice.

WARD NURSES

A named nurse, who plans your care on the ward.

PHYSIOTHERAPIST

Gives you exercises to do after surgery.

PSYCHOLOGIST

Professional counselling can help you to deal with decisions about treatment, depression and anxiety, and family issues.

SOCIAL WORKER

Can help solve practical difficulties, including transport, childcare and financial issues.

YOU REALLY NEED TO KNOW

◆ Your whole life changes when you are diagnosed with a life-threatening disease such as breast cancer, and the care you receive needs to address as many of your needs as possible.

◆ Breast lumps that might be cancer need to be investigated urgently, i.e. within three weeks.

◆ You have the right to ask for a second opinion, and you do not have to make any decisions until the diagnosis is definite.

The holistic approach

Principles of treatment

Treating breast cancer has three aims: to remove the primary tumour, to reduce the chance that the cancer will return in the breast or the armpit (local recurrence), and to reduce the chance that cancer will establish secondaries elsewhere in the body (distant spread).

Local treatment consists of surgery and radiotherapy. It is aimed at the lump and the lymph nodes in the armpit. Treatment additional to surgery is called adjuvant therapy, and consists of combinations of radiotherapy, chemotherapy and hormone therapy. Chemotherapy and hormone therapy are also called systemic treatment, because they affect the whole body, not just the local area, killing any cancer cells that have spread to sites beyond the breast and axilla. Even when there is no obvious distant spread, there may be micrometastasis, which is spread that is too small to be detected.

Your treatment plan

The treatment you receive will depend on your diagnosis. You may be offered a choice of operations, a combination of surgery and radiotherapy, or a combination of surgery and systemic treatment.

For women with early invasive breast cancer, the survival rate has been shown to be the same with either breast conservation or modified radical mastectomy (see p. 42). Breast conservation, which consists of lumpectomy (removal of the lump only), axillary node clearance and radiotherapy, can be considered whatever your age. But it is not suitable for women who choose not to have radiotherapy or who prefer to have the whole breast removed for peace of mind.

Most treatments for advanced cancer involving the skin and muscles of the armpit, with or without

TYPES OF THERAPY

LOCAL TREATMENT	◆ surgery ◆ radiotherapy
ADJUVANT THERAPY	◆ radiotherapy (local) ◆ chemotherapy (systemic) ◆ hormone therapy (systemic)
LOCAL TREATMENT WITH ADJUVANT THERAPY	◆ surgery + radiotherapy
SYSTEMIC TREATMENT (MAY OR MAY NOT INCLUDE SURGERY)	◆ chemotherapy ◆ surgery + chemotherapy ◆ radiotherapy + chemotherapy ◆ surgery + radiotherapy + chemotherapy ◆ hormone therapy ◆ surgery + hormone therapy ◆ surgery + hormone therapy + chemotherapy ◆ surgery + radiotherapy + hormone therapy ◆ surgery + radiotherapy + chemotherapy + hormone therapy

YOU REALLY NEED TO KNOW

◆ Treatment is aimed at the breast lump, the lymph nodes and distant disease.

◆ The most likely treatment for early breast cancer is surgery to remove the primary tumour.

◆ Treatment can be any combination of surgery, radiotherapy, chemotherapy or hormone therapy.

metastatic spread, include systemic therapy. For pre-menopausal women, this is usually chemotherapy and for older women it is commonly hormone therapy.

Principles of treatment

Surgical treatment

✓ Lumpectomy is a good option for some women, who often make a quicker recovery than those who have a mastectomy.

✗ Lumpectomy is not a good choice for women with very large tumours, as it would leave one breast much smaller than the other.

✓ If lumpectomy is not an option for you, you will be offered a mastectomy.

Surgery aims to remove as much cancerous tissue as possible from the breast. It is usually the first treatment for breast cancer and most women will have at least one operation during the course of their disease.

Lumpectomy

Studies have shown that for smaller tumours, a less extensive operation that removes the tumour but leaves most of the remaining breast tissue intact is as effective as removing the entire breast. Surgery that saves part of the breast is described as conservative and, although it is not suitable in all cases, many women have been spared the trauma of losing a breast.

In a lumpectomy, also called a partial mastectomy, the surgeon removes the lump plus a margin of breast tissue around it. The tissue that has been removed is sent to the laboratory where it is examined to check that the margins are clear of cancer. The operation is done under general anaesthetic, and you may be able to go

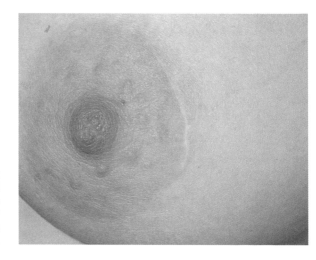

Depending on breast size, and the size and site of the tumour, the cosmetic result of lumpectomy can be very good.

home the same day. If not, you will only be in hospital for a few days. There will be a small scar where the incision was made, and you will have stitches, possibly a tube to drain blood and fluids and a dressing, which will be removed once healing is under way.

If the tumour lies directly below the nipple, lumpectomy includes removal of both the nipple and the areola, which leaves the breast mound but no nipple. If there is more than one tumour in the breast, or if the tumour is quite advanced, conservative surgery is not an option for you.

In most cases, the lymph nodes in the armpit have to be sampled through a separate incision, so if you have a lumpectomy you will usually require two incisions. You should receive radiotherapy to the breast (and sometimes also to the armpit) to reduce the chance of local recurrence.

Radical mastectomy

An operation in which the whole breast is removed is called a mastectomy, and there are three different types. The oldest is called radical mastectomy, but is hardly ever used now. Radical mastectomy—which is, as its name suggests, the most extensive form of mastectomy—involves removal of the entire breast including the skin and nipple, the nodes from the armpit, and the fat and muscles of the chest wall (the pectoralis muscles). This leaves only the ribcage covered by skin, and a very long scar. It weakens the arm because some of the muscles are removed. If you are offered a radical mastectomy, you may want to ask for a second opinion as advances in treatment mean it is rarely necessary to have such a major operation.

Surgical treatment

Surgical treatment

Modified radical mastectomy

This is less extensive and less mutilating than radical mastectomy. The breast, some of the lymph nodes and the smaller of the two chest muscles are removed. It leaves the pectoralis major muscle, which gives a better shape to the chest, and allows normal arm movement. Modified radical mastectomy is very commonly used in treating breast cancer.

Total mastectomy

Total mastectomy, also called simple mastectomy, involves removal of the breast alone. It does not always include axillary node clearance, although some nodes may be removed to look for cancer (called sampling). The chest muscles are not removed.

What to expect

Mastectomy is a major operation, and you will be in hospital for between five and 10 days. After the operation you will feel tender and bruised around the wound, and

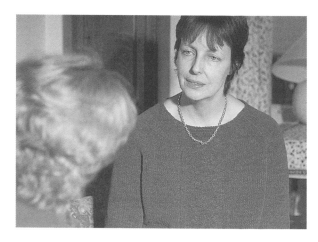

It can be very helpful to talk to someone who has been through breast surgery before finally deciding on the best treatment for you.

your shoulder might feel stiff. During some mastectomies, the surgeon inserts a drain. This is a small tube to remove fluid that may otherwise collect behind the stitches. The drain is usually removed between three and five days after the operation. Your stitches may be taken out while you are still in hospital, or you may have to go back for an outpatient appointment.

Deciding on surgery

Before deciding on surgery, make sure you know all the facts. Discuss your options with your consultant and other members of the team. Find out if the hospital can put you in touch with another breast cancer patient, or contact one of the voluntary organizations (see p. 78). Talking to someone who has been through breast surgery may help you to decide what is best for you. This is a good stage to talk about your options after the operation because what you choose now can limit your choices later. When deciding what type of surgery is best, you and your doctor need to go through the implications for reconstruction (see p. 48) and adjuvant therapy (see p.50).

Sentinel node mapping

Surgery to the axilla (see p. 44) can increase the risk of the operation but because it is important to know whether the lymph nodes contain cancer or not, a procedure called "sentinel node mapping" is sometimes carried out. During initial breast surgery, a radioactive dye is injected into the lymphatic vessels that lead to the axilla. The first node found to contain dye is removed and immediately examined under a microscope. If it is negative for cancer, no further surgery is required in this area, but if it is positive more nodes need to be removed.

3

YOU REALLY NEED TO KNOW

◆ You need time and support, in the form of advice and counselling, before making a final decision on the type of operation.

◆ It is important to be fully informed of all the advantages and disadvantages of the options open to you.

◆ Talk about reconstructive surgery with your doctor before you decide to go ahead with any operation.

Surgical treatment

43

Surgical treatment

Treating the axilla does not prevent breast cancer from spreading, but it is important in controlling local disease.

A diagnosis of breast cancer during pregnancy does not always mean the pregnancy must be terminated.

Some types of chemotherapy can be given in the last three months of pregnancy for the treatment of advanced, aggressive breast cancer.

Hormone therapy is never offered to pregnant women who have breast cancer.

Treating the axilla

Removing the lymph nodes of the axilla (armpit) makes it possible to see exactly how many are involved, and at what level. If most of the lymph nodes are involved, there is a higher chance of the cancer growing back in the armpit after surgery. This is called local recurrence and is difficult to treat. Up to 40 percent of women with invasive breast cancer have involved axillary nodes.

Axillary nodes are removed as part of a mastectomy. If they are removed as part of a lumpectomy, the surgeon makes a separate incision to remove them. In some cases, the surgeon carries out sentinel node mapping (see p. 43) so that he or she does not have to remove a large number of nodes unnecessarily. Removing the nodes doesn't stop the cancer spreading, but it does help to control the cancer in the axillary area.

REMOVING THE AXILLARY NODES

Axillary nodes are usually removed as part of a mastectomy. In axillary node clearance all the nodes are removed. If only a few are removed, to see if cancer is present, this is called sampling.

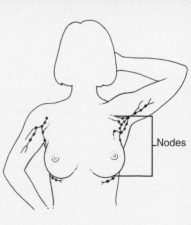

Nodes

Results of axillary surgery

Apart from the surgical scars, there is usually very little physical change after surgery. Sometimes, the skin of the armpit and the inside of the arm goes numb or tingly, and the arm on that side may swell as a result of fluid build up (or lymphoedema, see p. 47). This is more likely if all the nodes are removed or if you have a combination of surgery and radiotherapy to the axilla.

BREAST CANCER IN PREGNANCY

◆ Breast cancer occurs in fewer than three pregnancies in every 10,000. The diagnosis is made in the usual way, although the normal breast changes in pregnancy may make feeling a lump more difficult. Because of the possible effects on the developing fetus, treatment is slightly different.

◆ In the first six months, the standard treatment is modified radical mastectomy. Conservative treatment is not offered because radiation can harm the developing fetus, and the chance of the cancer recurring in lumpectomy without radiotherapy is up to 40 percent.

◆ There are a few more options if the diagnosis of breast cancer is made in the third trimester (the last three months of pregnancy). If the pregnancy is close to its end, treatment can be delayed by a week or two, or the baby may be delivered early. If the pregnancy is not so advanced, conservative surgery to remove the lump and axillary lymph nodes may be done straight away and radiotherapy and any other adjuvant therapy delayed until after the baby is born.

YOU REALLY NEED TO KNOW

◆ If the axillary lymph nodes are involved you will need treatment to this area.

◆ Removing all the involved lymph nodes from the axilla reduces the chance of local recurrence.

◆ Pregnant women who have breast cancer do not have to terminate the pregnancy, but in some cases delivery may be induced early.

◆ The type of treatment offered to a pregnant woman who has breast cancer depends on the stage of her pregnancy.

Surgical treatment

Surgical treatment

SELF-HELP

Taking something comforting like a photo can help you feel better in hospital.

Make sure you have some change handy for small purchases and a phonecard for phone calls. Mobile phones are not usually allowed.

In the hospital

You will be admitted to hospital the day before your operation so all the necessary tests and paperwork can be completed. The nursing staff will ask some questions about your lifestyle and health, weigh you, and take your temperature and blood pressure. You will also be seen by a doctor, and may be able to talk to the anaesthetist.

By the time you are admitted, you should know exactly what operation you are going to have, but you will still need to sign a consent form giving your permission for the surgery. As the doctor goes through the consent form, ask about anything you do not understand.

You will be asked not to eat or drink anything from around midnight the night before your operation to reduce the chance of vomiting or choking while you are anaesthetized. You should not see, hear or feel anything while you are under general anaesthetic, and you will not

WHY YOU NEED A DRIP

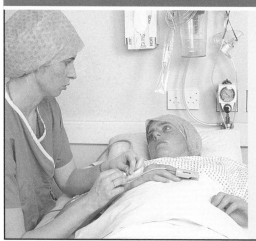

Soon after you are admitted to the ward for your operation the doctor will insert an intravenous cannula (also called a drip) into a vein, usually in your hand. This will be used for giving you fluids and medication after your operation, so that you do not need to have repeated injections. The cannula will be left in place until you are well enough to eat and drink again.

3

remember anything when you wake up, although you may feel drowsy and confused. The nursing staff can give you something if you feel sick.

After the operation

You will be encouraged to get out of bed as soon as possible. There is no need to be in any pain, so ask for painkillers if you find you need them. At first, your arm movement will be restricted, but you will be given exercises to do to help this. Drains are usually taken out after three to five days and stitches within two weeks. The scar will heal in two to four weeks, and will fade in time.

Lymphoedema

After surgery to the lymph nodes or radiotherapy to the axilla, the flow of lymph may be blocked, and this can cause the arm to swell up (lymphoedema). Improved techniques have made this less common, but it does still occur, especially after extensive axillary surgery or a combination of surgery and radiotherapy to the axilla. Treatment includes massage to encourage lymph drainage, use of a mechanical pump to reduce swelling, exercise and raising the arm.

Other complications

The wound may feel hot for a couple of days. If it becomes infected it will be red and tender, and you may need antibiotics. If fluid builds up behind the stitches after the drain has been removed or if one was not used, it may need to be drained. Other complications that can occur after any operation are chest infection and a clot in a leg vein. Both can be prevented, or treated if they appear, but occasionally they can be serious.

**YOU REALLY
NEED TO KNOW**

◆ Surgical treatment for breast cancer is done under general anaesthetic.

◆ Any pain after surgery can be controlled very effectively with painkillers.

◆ There may be some complications after an operation, but most of these are not serious.

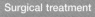

Surgical treatment

Reconstructive surgery

After a mastectomy, it is often possible to reconstruct the breast area to restore the contour and original appearance of the breast. No reconstruction will ever look or feel exactly like the natural breast, but using tissue from your own body, or a synthetic implant, the surgeon can create a breast that looks fine except under very close examination. Not all women want reconstruction, but if you think that it might make you feel more positive, ask if it is available in your case. It is not suitable for women with very advanced disease, nor for those whose cancer is actively spreading.

When is reconstruction done?

Reconstructive surgery can be done immediately (at the time the natural breast is removed), or later, when other treatment is completed. Some doctors prefer to wait for

WHAT HAPPENS IN A BREAST IMPLANT

The doctor inserts a temporary expanding implant under the mastectomy scar (there is no need for a second scar). Each week he or she injects more fluid into the implant and the skin gradually stretches (expands) until there is enough space underneath to insert the permanent implant. The permanent implant is made of silicone filled with saline fluid or silicone gel. The end result can look and feel very natural, but there is a risk of your body reacting to the foreign material, causing a build up of fibrous tissue which makes the breast feel hard. The other disadvantages are that it is done in stages, takes time and requires weekly visits. There is also a chance that the implant may leak.

two years, as reconstruction can make it harder to detect any recurrence. The advantages of immediate reconstruction are that you need only one major operation, and therefore only one general anaesthetic. Some women also find it less traumatic to wake up with a breast mound already in place. The disadvantages are that the actual operation takes longer to perform than mastectomy alone and there is a slight increase in the number of complications that may occur, which may mean delaying further treatment.

Waiting until all local and adjuvant therapy (see p. 50) is completed makes sense to many women. Another advantage is that it gives you time to adjust to your new, altered body appearance, to consider all your options and to explore alternatives to surgery.

Different types of reconstruction

Reconstructive surgery cannot create a perfect replacement in a single operation. The new breast will look different, and it usually takes a couple more minor operations to complete. The surgeon can either use tissue from your own body (autologous tissue) or an implant. Suitable tissue can be taken from the muscles of the back, stomach, buttocks or outside of the thigh. When using the back or stomach muscle, the surgeon cuts a flap of tissue, still attached to its original blood supply, and sews it into place over the mastectomy site. The back muscle has a good blood supply, but leaves a visible scar and is not large enough to fill more than a C-cup bra. It also limits arm and shoulder movement. The stomach muscle has more tissue available, but may not be suitable if you are overweight as it weakens the stomach wall and can lead to a hernia.

YOU REALLY NEED TO KNOW

◆ Reconstructive surgery can be done at the same time as a mastectomy.

◆ Choosing delayed reconstruction gives you time to adjust to your new shape, and to consider all your possible options.

◆ The surgeon can reconstruct the breast using tissue taken from your own body, especially back or stomach muscles.

◆ Breast implants can give very good results, but some women's bodies do not accept the silicone that is used in implants.

Reconstructive surgery

Adjuvant treatment

The real problem with breast cancer is that, even after an operation, it can recur in the breast (local spread) and can also spread to other parts of the body (distant spread), where it forms secondary tumours. Treatment that is given after surgery to reduce the chance of spread is called adjuvant treatment. Even when there is no evidence of local spread, the seeds of distant spread may be present but undetectable. Adjuvant treatment aims to eradicate these seeds so no secondaries develop. As this is not always a realistic goal, the second aim is to delay recurrence of the cancer. Adjuvant therapy may take the form of radiotherapy, chemotherapy or hormone therapy.

Who has adjuvant treatment?

As with most aspects of this complex disease, there is no simple answer as to who should have adjuvant treatment. When deciding whether or not to give it, doctors try to predict the likelihood that the patient's tumour will recur. It is impossible to know for sure how a cancer will behave, but there are some factors that indicate that recurrence or distant spread is more likely. These include the invasiveness of the tumour (in situ tumours do not need adjuvant therapy), the size of the tumour, the number of lymph nodes involved, whether the tumour is sensitive to the hormones oestrogen and progesterone (measured using hormone receptor tests) and the aggressiveness of the tumour.

Which type of therapy?

The exact type of adjuvant therapy recommended will depend on three things—whether you have had your menopause or are still having periods, whether the

3

NEO-ADJUVANT THERAPY

Therapy can be used to shrink a cancer before surgery. This is known as neo-adjuvant therapy. It makes surgery technically easier and perhaps more effective. Also, giving therapy such as chemotherapy before surgery can show whether or not the cancer responds to those drugs. If so, they may be useful after the operation as well.

YOU REALLY NEED TO KNOW

◆ Chemotherapy, radiotherapy and hormone therapy are the most commonly used types of adjuvant therapy.

◆ Adjuvant therapy has its own risks and side effects.

◆ In situ cancer does not need treatment with adjuvant therapy.

tumour had hormone receptors on it when it was tested and, when there is more than one option to be considered, your own feelings and preferences.

Radiotherapy
In radiotherapy high-energy radiation (similar to X-rays) is used to treat disease. When radiotherapy is used to treat breast cancer, it consists of directing beams of radiation at the cancer site to kill any cancer cells left behind after surgery. In the past, all women with breast cancer used to receive radiotherapy but doctors now select those who will benefit most to avoid irradiating women unnecessarily.

When is radiotherapy given?
Conservative therapy for early disease consists of radiotherapy given after lumpectomy and axillary node clearance. This gives the same results as modified radical mastectomy. In more advanced cancer, when the tumour is larger, or there is node involvement or spread to the skin and chest wall, radiotherapy is given after mastectomy and axillary clearance.

Adjuvant treatment

Where is the radiation directed?

After a lumpectomy, the radiotherapy will be directed at the remaining breast tissue. With modern techniques, it is possible to limit the amount of radiation that reaches the ribs, lungs and heart, although small doses will pass through healthy tissue on the way to the cancer site. After a mastectomy, the chest wall will be irradiated, and if there is node involvement or a strong chance that the cancer will recur, the axilla will also be treated, as will the area above the collar bone, where other lymph nodes are situated.

Radiotherapy is also used to treat local recurrence at the original site or in the armpit, and in late stage breast cancer to try to shrink a tumour that is too big to remove.

How is radiotherapy given?

An average course of radiotherapy consists of treatment five days a week for five or six weeks, starting approximately a month after surgery, when you are able

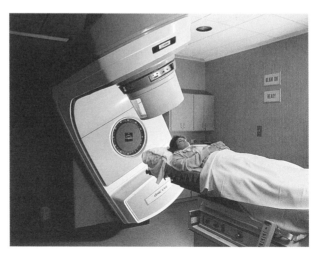

To make sure you receive the right dose of radiation in the correct place, you have to lie in the same position each time (usually lying down with your arm above your head). You need to lie absolutely still while the radiation is being given.

to move your arm and shoulder again. You will visit the hospital each day and return home afterwards. Treatment takes a few minutes—the actual exposure to radiation lasts only about five minutes, but it also takes a little while to position you correctly.

Side effects of radiotherapy

While you are having the treatment you may feel very tired, but you will not lose the hair on your head and you are unlikely to feel nauseous. The main short-term side effect is a skin reaction. The area may feel "sunburned", and become dry and scaly or itchy. The skin often goes darker, but this is not permanent. You may also get some little red marks caused by small blood vessels bursting.

You can try to prevent problems by careful skin care. This includes gentle washing, avoiding the use of soap, talcum powder and skin lotion, and not exposing the area to the sun. You may be given a mild steroid cream or a petroleum jelly dressing to apply. Most skin reactions settle within a few weeks of the end of treatment.

The long-term side effects of radiotherapy are more troublesome, but are rare. Approximately 12 percent of women who have axillary surgery and radiotherapy develop lymphoedema, or swelling of the arm (see p. 47). Tell your doctor if you notice any puffiness or swelling so that it can be treated as soon as possible.

Occasionally, radiotherapy affects the surrounding healthy tissues. This can lead to problems such as pneumonitis, which is an inflammation of the lungs. It is very rare, but if it does develop it causes shortness of breath and a dry cough. Another possible problem is damage to the ribs, which may be weakened by radiotherapy and, very occasionally, can break.

YOU REALLY NEED TO KNOW

◆ Radiotherapy kills cancer cells with high-energy radiation.

◆ Not everybody who has breast cancer needs radiotherapy.

◆ Radiotherapy has few side effects, compared with chemotherapy.

Adjuvant treatment

Systemic therapy

✓ Chemotherapy is particularly effective in pre-menopausal women.

✓ In some cases, chemotherapy is offered before surgery to try and shrink the tumour so that less extensive surgery is then needed.

Systemic therapy is treatment that circulates throughout the whole body looking for cancer cells. It aims to improve the survival rate in women whose cancer has already spread beyond the primary tumour.

If you have had your menopause and your cancer has hormone receptors, hormone therapy is generally recommended. If it had no hormone receptors, chemotherapy is usually recommended. Pre-menopausal women are usually recommended to have chemotherapy.

Chemotherapy

Treatment of cancer with cytotoxic drugs (drugs designed to find and destroy cancer cells) is known as chemotherapy. Side effects occur because some healthy cells are sacrificed along the way. Cancer drugs need to be toxic to be effective, but those that are generally used for breast cancer are some of the least harmful.

In pre-menopausal women the most common type of chemotherapy is a combination of three drugs—

CHEMOTHERAPY DRUG COMBINATIONS

◆ Neoadjuvant (before surgery or radiotherapy to shrink the tumour)
FAC; ECF; MMM

◆ Adjuvant (after surgery where there is thought to be minimal disease, i.e. as an insurance)
CMF; AC or EC

◆ Metastatic disease
Any of the above but also taxanes, herceptin and navelbine

Key: A = adriamycin
E = epirubicin
C = cyclophosphamide or cisplatinum
F = 5-fluorouracil
MMM = methotrexate and mitomycin
C and mitozantrone

cyclophosphamide, methotrexate and 5-fluorouracil (CMF). The cyclophosphamide is usually given as a tablet every day for two weeks, and the other two drugs are given by injection or through a drip inserted into a vein in your arm (see p. 46). If you have a drip, you may need to stay in hospital overnight, but usually you can have your chemotherapy as an out-patient.

Post-menopausal women with tumours negative for hormone receptors (see p. 58) are usually given a different chemotherapy, which contains a drug called adriamycin.

The timing of chemotherapy varies, but it is usually given for six months in total (four for adriamycin-containing combinations), with a series of treatments once a month. Traditionally, chemotherapy was given after surgery and radiotherapy, but ongoing research is looking at alternatives, such as giving half the chemotherapy, pausing for radiotherapy, then completing the treatment with more chemotherapy.

Very high-dose chemotherapy

Some cancers may respond to very high-dose chemotherapy, and if this is the case, you may be offered a bone marrow transplant. This means that some of your bone marrow will be removed before the chemotherapy starts, stored for you and then put back after chemotherapy. The same can be done with stem cells (the immature cells that divide to make new blood cells). Stem cells can be harvested from the blood or bone marrow, and because they have not been affected by the chemotherapy, when they are returned to the body they can still produce healthy blood cells. Whether this treatment is beneficial in breast cancer is still under review, so do discuss it with your doctor.

YOU REALLY NEED TO KNOW

◆ Systemic treatment is aimed at metastatic disease—cancer that has spread to other parts of the body.

◆ All breast cancers with lymph node involvement need adjuvant therapy of some sort.

◆ Late stage cancer may be treated with palliative chemotherapy only. This relieves the pain and slows progress of the disease but does not cure the cancer.

Systemic therapy

Systemic therapy

✓ New treatments have made nausea and vomiting much less of a problem than they used to be.

✓ Mouth ulcers and infections can be prevented by careful tooth brushing and regular use of a mouthwash.

Side effects of chemotherapy

The most dangerous side effect is temporary suppression of the immune system, a serious problem for about one in 20 women. It occurs because the chemotherapy damages the bone marrow where the blood cells are made. If you do not have enough white cells you cannot fight infection, so your blood will be tested before each treatment and if your white cell count is too low, your chemotherapy dose will be adjusted or delayed. Red blood cells are also affected, and you may need a transfusion to top up your levels.

Nausea and vomiting are very common. If this happens, future doses will be reduced as far as possible without interfering with their effectiveness. There are also new, effective treatments to prevent nausea. Chemotherapy leaves most people feeling drained but energy levels usually return to normal about a month after the end of chemotherapy.

Some women also find they put on weight. Get advice on modifying your diet, and, if you feel up to it, join an enjoyable exercise programme to help you feel better and prevent you gaining weight.

Fertility problems

With chemotherapy your periods can become irregular or stop. In younger women, menstruation tends to start again once treatment has ended, but about 40 percent of women will not menstruate again. After the age of 40, you are more likely become infertile after chemotherapy. Some women experience menopausal symptoms, such as vaginal dryness and hot flushes. Simple lubricants may help with vaginal dryness, while hot flushes tend to disappear after a while.

LOSING YOUR HAIR

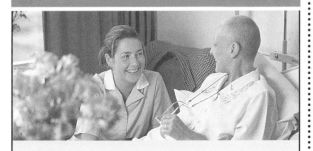

Hair loss is a distressing side effect that begins about three weeks after the start of chemotherapy. Not everybody loses all their hair, and you may find yours only gets thinner. The psychological effect of losing your hair can be traumatic, especially after losing a breast, but knowing it is not permanent and preparing for it in advance by buying a wig (see p. 67) helps many women cope better.

Preparing for chemotherapy

All these unpleasant possibilities, combined with the stress of having cancer, can be taxing emotionally and psychologically. You can prepare for the physical strain by getting plenty of rest, eating well, and taking vitamin and mineral supplements.

Emotionally you may find it helps to take the initiative and to think of chemotherapy as a powerful weapon you have chosen to use to fight the cancer. This may make the side effects a little more bearable. But feeling depressed or anxious is normal and nothing to be ashamed of. Asking for help is not always easy; talk to someone else on the team if your specialist seems too busy to spare the time.

YOU REALLY NEED TO KNOW

◆ The most serious side effect of chemotherapy is weakening of the immune system, which increases the risk of infection.

◆ Other side effects can be rather unpleasant but are not dangerous.

◆ Most side effects of chemotherapy are not permanent.

Systemic therapy

Systemic therapy

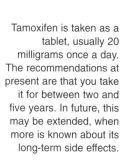
Hormone therapy

The growth of some breast cancers is influenced by hormones, especially oestrogen. A test can be done on a sample of the cancer to see if the cells contain what are called hormone receptors (oestrogen receptors and progesterone receptors). If the cancer cells do contain one or both types of receptor it is a "receptor-positive" cancer and hormone therapy has a high chance of success. In general, receptor-positive cancers have a better outlook than receptor-negative cancers. If the cancer cells are receptor-negative, hormone therapy will not work, and your doctor will recommend chemotherapy.

The most common hormone therapy used in breast cancer is the drug tamoxifen, which blocks oestrogen. It works best for post-menopausal women with hormone receptor-positive tumours. For this group, it may be the only adjuvant therapy needed.

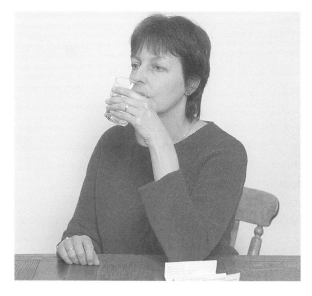

Tamoxifen is taken as a tablet, usually 20 milligrams once a day. The recommendations at present are that you take it for between two and five years. In future, this may be extended, when more is known about its long-term side effects.

Tamoxifen may also benefit pre-menopausal women, although to a lesser extent than women over 50. This is why it is used following chemotherapy in treating younger women. Although tamoxifen cures fewer breast cancers in women under 50, it lengthens the time before possible recurrence. Younger women get less benefit from tamoxifen because they tend to have hormone receptor-negative breast cancer, and because their ovaries are still producing oestrogen.

What are the side effects?

The side effects of tamoxifen are relatively rare and mild. Because of its effect on oestrogen, it can cause menopausal symptoms, such as hot flushes, vaginal dryness, vaginal discharge and weight gain. There may be a slightly increased chance of getting a deep vein thrombosis (a blood clot in your calf) and there is also a slightly increased risk of developing cataracts (damage to the lens of the eye that blurs vision).

The most serious effect of tamoxifen is the increased risk of developing endometrial cancer (cancer of the lining of the womb). Women who take hormone replacement therapy (HRT) share this risk, but the risks need to be weighed against the benefits. The chances of a woman with breast cancer developing endometrial cancer after taking tamoxifen are much smaller than the chances of her developing a second breast cancer if she does not take tamoxifen. It is reassuring to know that you can have check-ups for endometrial cancer; these include a yearly examination and regular ultrasound scans of the womb. You should also watch out for any abnormal or very heavy periods and report them to your doctor as soon as possible.

YOU REALLY NEED TO KNOW

◆ Hormone therapy improves survival rate and can cure some breast cancers.

◆ Tamoxifen increases your risk of endometrial cancer threefold, but greatly reduces the risk of developing a second breast cancer.

Systemic therapy

Systemic therapy

Positive side effects

Tamoxifen also has beneficial side effects, such as protecting against osteoporosis (thinning of the bones) and heart disease. The biggest advantage is that it halves your chances of getting breast cancer in your other breast. Ongoing trials are attempting to find out whether tamoxifen can prevent breast cancer from developing in the first place.

Removal of the ovaries

Surgery to remove the ovaries (oophorectomy), or radiation to destroy them (ovarian ablation), changes the levels of hormones in the body, which in turn has an effect on how breast cancer behaves. Oophorectomy was first used to treat breast cancer in the 1940s, but was performed less and less as chemotherapy was developed. Researchers are now looking at whether

---

GENETIC RESEARCH AND BREAST CANCER

The ERB-B2 mutation

Research is currently uncovering genetic changes that play a part in the development of breast cancer. For example, about 20 to 30 percent of breast cancers are associated with what is known as the ERB-B2 gene mutation. A certain sequence on a gene, given the name ERB-B2, stimulates cancer cells to grow. The recently developed drug herceptin helps to block the effects of the ERB-B2 gene, making use of the body's own immune system.

oophorectomy can be used instead of, or as well as, chemotherapy. An injection of an ovary-suppressing drug, such as goserelin, is sometimes used to induce a temporary, reversible menopause in younger, pre-menopausal women.

The disadvantage of oophorectomy is that it causes an immediate menopause. Women who are at very high risk of recurrence may choose to give up their ability to have children to improve their chances of a cure.

Prophylactic mastectomy

In any disease, prevention is better than cure. This is especially true when you are dealing with life-threatening cancer, and there is a lot of research aimed at breast cancer prevention, also called prophylaxis.

Women who are at very high risk of breast cancer may consider having a double mastectomy to try and prevent it developing. This is a dramatic and irreversible step, and the decision takes time to make, but if you have lost more than one close family member to breast cancer or tests show that you have a gene that carries a high risk of breast cancer (see p. 17), and you are very worried about developing the disease yourself, having a prophylactic mastectomy may give you some peace of mind. Also, if you are at high risk and your breasts are not easy to examine or your mammograms are not easy to interpret—perhaps because your breasts are very small—you may want to consider having the operation.

The decision to have this drastic surgery should never be made in a hurry. Take six months to go through all your options, get counselling, and discuss the pros and cons fully with your partner, family and friends before finally deciding to go ahead.

YOU REALLY NEED TO KNOW

◆ Oophorectomy improves survival rate in women under 50.

◆ Oophorectomy leaves you infertile.

◆ Tamoxifen prevents disability and death by protecting against osteoporosis and heart disease.

◆ You can still get breast cancer even after a prophylactic mastectomy.

Systemic therapy

Chapter

4

LIVING WITH CANCER

Looking and feeling good   64

After treatment   68

Talking to children   72

Palliative care   74

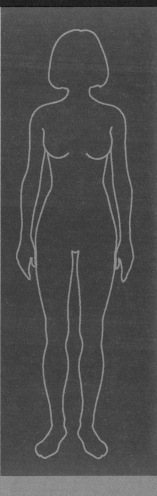

Looking and feeling good

✓ After a radical mastectomy the arm on the affected side will be permanently weakened because the muscles of the chest wall have been removed, but exercise will improve mobility.

✓ Try to exercise for short periods every day rather than longer, less frequent sessions.

EVERYDAY EXERCISES

After surgery you will need to exercise your arm and shoulder to get full movement back. Exercises will usually be recommended by the physiotherapist in hospital as early as the second day after surgery. Follow medical advice and do not try to do too much too soon. The exercises illustrated below can safely be done at home.

◆ Rotate your shoulder on the affected side in a circular motion, leaving your arm hanging by your side.

◆ Rest your elbow on the affected side on a firm surface and brush your hair.

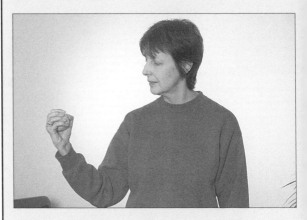

◆ Hold a soft ball in your hand on the affected side (above) and squeeze and release it a few times, increasing the number of times as your strength returns.

◆ Practise doing up your bra, clasping your hands behind your back and then stretching them out sideways.

◆ Hold a large towel with one hand over your shoulder and the other behind your waist. Dry your back using a series of long, slow, diagonal movements, then change hands.

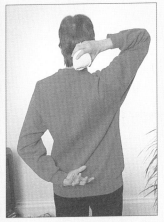

◆ Hold a bean bag in one hand, lift it and drop it behind your back (left), catching it with your other hand. Repeat with the other arm. You can make a bean bag out of a sock.

◆ Hold either end of a rope hanging over a door. Sit with the door between your knees. Pull the rope with one hand so the other arm goes up, then pull that arm down, and so on.

◆ It is important to exercise your arm and shoulder after surgery so that you regain full movement.

◆ Always follow medical advice and do not try to do too much too soon.

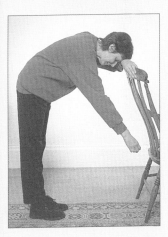

◆ Lean on the back of a chair, with your forehead resting on your good arm (left). Let your weak arm hang loosely, then swing it forwards and backwards, side to side, and round and round.

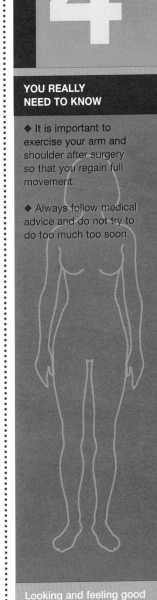

Looking and feeling good

Looking and feeling good

When deciding whether to wear a wig or a prosthesis the best advice is to explore all the options and choose the one that suits your lifestyle.

Breast prostheses

Worrying about your appearance and wanting to look as good as you can are normal feelings. Some women think they are being vain if they ask about prostheses or wigs during treatment for cancer. But self-image and emotional well-being are important, and if wearing a wig or an attractive outfit makes you feel better, it is worth it, especially as there is evidence that your state of mind plays an important role in the outcome of your treatment.

A breast prosthesis is a false breast, which may or may not have a nipple. If you have decided against reconstruction, or are still in the process of making up your mind, you may want to find out about prostheses.

CHOOSING THE PROSTHESIS FOR YOU

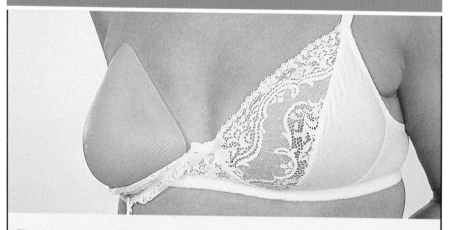

There are many different shapes, colours and sizes of prosthesis available, as well as a variety of nipples. Breast forms can also be custom made. Breast prostheses and fitting are free of charge for patients treated on the NHS, but not all private health insurance schemes contribute to the cost of prostheses.

All women who have had a mastectomy are strongly recommended to try out a properly fitted, weighted breast form. Before leaving hospital, you should have had the opportunity to wear a much lighter, temporary prosthesis, while your scar was healing.

Within four to six weeks of surgery you will be ready to be fitted for a permanent prosthesis. Prostheses are made from silicone, and have the same weight and feel as a natural breast. They last for two to four years. Silicone is waterproof and can be worn safely during most activities.

Some prostheses can be attached directly to the skin with an adhesive strip. Others slip into a pocket in a special bra, which may be soft-cup or underwired. The bras are made with wider straps and a larger underband than regular bras, and are available in several different styles and colours.

You will be able to wear most styles of clothing. Special swimming costumes are available, although you may still be able to wear an ordinary one. Someone on your team should be able to give you information about where you can go for all the supplies you need.

Wigs

If your treatment includes chemotherapy, you may lose some or all of your hair. It is a good idea to think about what you would like to do before this happens. Some women find it boosts their morale to have an attractive wig ready before chemotherapy starts—perhaps even to radically change their hair colour or style. Your breast care nurse or someone else on your team will be able to advise you on where to get one. Alternatively, you might like to experiment with different hats and scarves.

YOU REALLY NEED TO KNOW

◆ Self-image and emotional well-being are important, so do not be afraid to ask for information about prostheses and wigs.

◆ Prostheses are available in different materials and skin tones and in a wide range of shapes and sizes. They can also be custom made.

Looking and feeling good

After treatment

Local recurrence is most common in conserved breast tissue after a lumpectomy. In two percent of women it occurs in the lymph nodes in the armpit.

Recurrence in your other breast, in your scar or elsewhere is more serious than local recurrence and means that the cancer has spread.

Once treatment is over you may be surprised to feel rather lost—the period of activity and doing something about your illness is gone and you no longer have regular contact with all the familiar medical staff. You may feel unsupported, at the very time when you are adjusting to the physical and psychological changes that have taken place. It's normal to feel sad for the loss of the person you were before your illness. Take all the time you need to come to terms with the fact that the changes are permanent. Many women find it helps to have an outlet for their feelings. This could be your GP, a psychologist, a religious counsellor, or a support group (see p. 78).

Your sexual self

For many people sex is a very important part of their relationship, yet it is one that is rarely talked about openly and candidly. But when a serious illness affects one

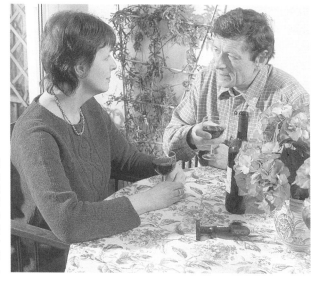

Many women worry that their partner will find them less attractive after breast surgery, but a lot of couples find that the experience of tackling breast cancer together strengthens the bond between them.

partner, it is vital to talk. Getting sex started again after a major life change such as treatment for breast cancer is never easy and may be awkward and embarrassing at first. If you have had a mastectomy or chemotherapy you may feel sensitive about your changed appearance.

Set aside a time to talk to your partner and to listen to what he has to say. You may not feel ready for full intercourse, but try to be specific about what you are prepared to do. Often a cuddle and a hug will be enough to bring you closer at first and if you have discussed it in advance will not cause distrust or guilt if things go no farther at the time. Gradually you will feel ready to move on to a wider range of sexual activities.

Accepting the new you

In time, you will come to accept your new shape, and feel proud of what you have achieved. Your choices about reconstruction, prostheses and clothing are all part of the process of reaffirming yourself as a woman. Each individual experience is unique, but the strength and support gained from sharing your concerns with others in the same position, or with a counsellor, can speed up the recovery and healing processes.

What about recurrence?

When surgery and any adjuvant treatment are completed, your cancer may be in remission. You will be relieved, but now comes a different type of stress.

You and your doctor need to be on the lookout for recurrence, especially in the next five years. You need to make a clear plan for follow-up and review, with regular appointments for the first two years, and then a yearly check-up, including a mammogram and a chest X-ray.

After treatment

After treatment

Research shows that your state of mind may play a role in boosting your body's natural defences against cancer.

Some alternative therapies are known to be beneficial, but others may have a damaging effect on the outcome of conventional treatment or may even be dangerous.

What about support?

You should know who to phone if you are concerned about anything. Having this structure in place can be reassuring, but many women experience periods of extreme anxiety and fear that their cancer has returned. If these feelings become overwhelming, you may need help from your doctor. Anxiety and depression can be treated with counselling and anti-depressant drugs, so do say at once if you are feeling low or are unusually tearful or irritable, if your appetite has changed or if you are having difficulty sleeping.

Living your life

Treatment for breast cancer can be uncomfortable and exhausting. Looking forward and making plans to enjoy life once your treatment is over will help to make the

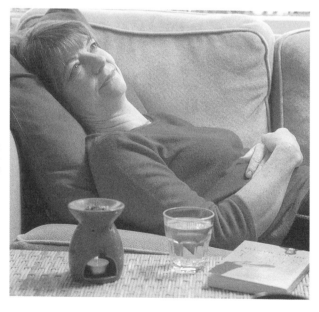

In future, all breast cancer centres may offer a range of complementary and alternative therapies alongside the traditional treatments. Until then you can find out what is available in your area from your doctor's surgery or a breast cancer support group.

discomfort easier to bear. It is important to look after yourself and to get involved in activities that you find rewarding. Many women find that their attitude to life has changed—for example, little problems may no longer seem so important. You might decide to do something you have always wanted to do but never got round to or you may simply want to get back to your normal routine as quickly as possible. Whatever your choices, give yourself time to adjust to this new phase of life. Breast cancer is a major crisis in any woman's life, and physical and emotional recovery take time.

Complementary therapies

Therapies that "complement" conventional medicine and can be used with it, such as homeopathy, massage and aromatherapy, are known as complementary. Alternative therapies, such as herbalism, are not usually used alongside conventional medicine. You may be interested in finding out whether any of these therapies suit you. But remember when exploring the options that it is important—even if you are feeling disappointed or fed up with your current treatment programme—to let your specialist or the breast care nurse know which other therapies you want to try.

The modern approach to cancer treatment is for doctors to encourage any complementary therapies that have a positive impact on the patient. Therapies being used include visualization techniques, meditation and relaxation, acupuncture and vitamin supplements. However, no responsible complementary or alternative practitioner would ever advise you to stop all other treatments or claim to offer a "cure" for cancer—it is illegal to make this claim in the UK.

YOU REALLY NEED TO KNOW

◆ Talking about your experiences and worries will help you to come to terms with them.

◆ There are breast cancer counsellors and support groups that can give you help and support when you need it.

◆ Not all alternative therapies are harmless, so get as much information and advice as possible before you try any different type of treatment.

After treatment

Talking to children

You may feel you want to protect your children by not telling them about your breast cancer for as long as possible, but you should avoid this temptation. Even young children know when something is wrong and if they are not told the truth they can feel isolated and more anxious. Children also have an amazing capacity for dealing with unpleasant facts.

When should I tell my children?

Talk to your children as soon as you have been diagnosed with breast cancer. The amount of detail you go into will depend on their ages and how easy you find it to talk about your cancer. Explain what is wrong and what your treatment will involve, including any possible side effects. You may find it easier to talk to your children individually at this stage.

Talk about your treatment

Keep your children informed as your treatment progresses, without going into too much detail. If you are going to have chemotherapy, for example, warn your children that your hair will fall out and tell them that it will grow back in time. Tell them also that you will be very tired while your treatment is happening, but try to spend time with them doing activities that are not too tiring, such as watching TV or playing board games.

Children's worries

You will need to be sensitive to your children's reactions. Younger children may worry that they have caused your cancer or that they might catch it. Reassure them that cancer is an illness that is not caused by anyone, neither is it catching. Remember, information is power.

PLAN WHAT YOU WILL SAY

Before you tell your children about your cancer, it may help to plan what you are going to say and how you will say it.

DO...

◆ Avoid medical terms—use language your children can easily understand.

◆ Listen to your children to find out how much information they can cope with at any one time.

◆ Be truthful—children know when you are hiding something from them.

◆ Correct any mistaken ideas they may have.

◆ Try to keep your home routine as normal as possible.

◆ Let your children's school know what is happening.

◆ Tell your children honestly how you feel.

◆ Remember it's OK to cry—for you and your children.

◆ Be prepared to repeat information and to answer questions as often as your children need.

◆ Stress the positive whenever you can.

◆ Use dolls and role play to explain the situation to a younger child.

◆ Contact a support group and get together with other families who are coping with cancer (see p. 78).

DON'T...

◆ Be afraid to say "I don't know."

◆ Hide your emotions—honesty is the best policy.

◆ Give children too many medical details.

◆ Push your children to talk if they are not ready.

◆ Make promises unless you are sure you can keep them.

YOU REALLY NEED TO KNOW

◆ Children have the right to know about things that affect the family—as cancer does.

◆ Teenagers may find it particularly hard to cope with their emotions when they are told.

◆ Some children may be afraid that they too will develop cancer.

◆ If you don't tell your children the truth they may learn it from someone else, or get misleading information from other sources.

Talking to children

73

Palliative care

In some cases, the breast cancer may recur and progress despite treatment. If that happens and a cure is no longer possible the objective of all treatment and support becomes the control of any symptoms you may develop. This is called palliative care, a branch of medicine that focuses on the quality of life for patients who cannot be cured. Palliative care aims to strike the right balance between trying to extend life at all costs and trying to make the end of a terminal illness as peaceful as possible.

Accepting the inevitable

Death and dying are not subjects that most of us feel comfortable talking or thinking about. Knowing that you have a life-threatening disease means you have probably thought more about it than others, but you may still find it difficult to talk about, especially to your loved ones. There comes a time for some women with breast cancer when everybody, from the patient to her family and the team looking after her, will need to adjust to the knowledge that the disease is now terminal.

Possible reactions

You may go through a number of different reactions. You may experience shock or disbelief; you may become very angry; you may be very frightened; some people even feel guilty (although nobody should); and some people just cannot take in the reality.

Coming to terms with your illness will take time. You may feel lonely and afraid along the way, and find that your priorities change with time, but it can help to share your fears with other breast cancer sufferers, a counsellor, and your family and friends. Having some

WHAT A HOSPICE CAN OFFER

Hospices can help with many aspects of your disease, from pain management to tips on preparing food and skincare after surgery. They also provide support and counselling, both to the patient and her family. You may want financial or legal advice to help you get your affairs in order, or to discuss your religious and spiritual needs. The hospice can help with all of these, more so than a general hospital, because staff have time and training to focus on the specific needs of cancer patients.

The old-fashioned view of hospices as places people go to die is fading, but you may still feel shocked if your doctor suggests you contact a hospice. The modern role of hospices includes caring for cancer patients at home as well as providing in-patient care.

YOU REALLY NEED TO KNOW

◆ Palliative care is provided by hospices, both for in-patients and for people living in their own homes.

◆ Most types of pain can be very well controlled using modern methods of pain-relief.

◆ Adjusting to the knowledge that your disease is terminal takes time, both for you and your family.

idea of how to handle the inevitable end and making plans helps both patients and their family and friends cope better. When everything is settled and everyone knows what you want, you may not need to talk about the subject ever again.

Controlling pain

Nowadays, really effective pain control can be achieved for the vast majority of patients. The most important message to remember is that most pain, whether mild or severe, short-term or long-term, can be well controlled and there is no need to suffer. If your doctor does not know what services are available locally, contact one of the organizations listed on p. 78 for advice.

Palliative care

Understanding the jargon

Many of the terms that you will meet when finding out more about breast cancer may be unfamiliar to you. This page gives definitions of the words you are most likely to come across.

ADJUVANT—treatment used in addition to surgery

AXILLA—the armpit

BENIGN—a tumour that grows in one place and does not spread to any other part of the body

BIOPSY—the removal of a piece of tissue from the body for examination under a microscope

CHEMOTHERAPY—the use of drugs to destroy cancer cells throughout the body

CYTOLOGY—the examination of cells under the microscope to look for evidence of disease

DYSPLASIA—abnormal cell growth

GENE—a piece of DNA that contains information that controls how cells behave

HORMONE—a chemical in the body that influences how cells and body systems work

HYPERPLASIA—overgrowth of cells

IN SITU—tumour growth that has not invaded any of the surrounding tissue

LUMPECTOMY—surgical removal of a breast lump

LYMPH NODE—part of the lymphatic system that becomes enlarged when affected by disease

LYMPHOEDEMA—swelling (for example of the arm) when lymph drainage becomes blocked, especially after radiotherapy

MALIGNANT—cancer that invades the surrounding tissue and other areas of the body

MAMMOGRAM—X-ray of the breast

MASTECTOMY—surgical removal of the breast

METASTASIS—spread of cancer from the primary site to a secondary site in the body

OOPHORECTOMY—surgical removal of the ovaries

PALLIATIVE TREATMENT—treating the symptoms of terminal disease in order to improve quality of life

PRIMARY CANCER—the original tumour before any spread took place

REMISSION—when a disease is present but not active, for example after treatment

SECONDARIES—tumours that grow as a result of spread from the primary (also called metastases)

SYSTEMIC—treatment that reaches all the systems of the body, not just the breast

TUMOUR—an abnormal growth or lump, which may be benign or malignant

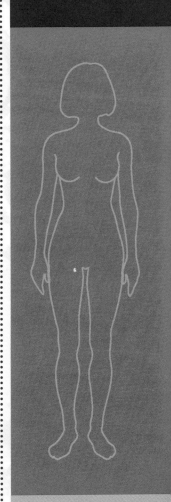

Understanding the jargon

Useful addresses

BREAKTHROUGH BREAST CANCER
6th Floor Kingsway House
103 Kingsway
London WC2B 6QX
Tel: 020 7405 5111
www.breakthrough.org.uk

BREAST CANCER CARE
210 New Kings Road
London SW6 4NZ
Tel: 020 7384 2984
Freephone helpline: 0808 800 6000
www.breastcancercare.org.uk

CANCERBACUP
3 Bath Place
Rivington Street
London EC2A 3JR
Information line: 020 7613 2121
Freephone: 0808 800 1234
Administration: 020 7696 9003
www.cancerbacup.org.uk

CANCERLINK
11–21 Northdown Street
London N1 9BN
Freephone helpline: 0808 808 0000

INSTITUTE FOR COMPLEMENTARY MEDICINE
PO Box 194
London SE16 1QZ
Tel: 020 7237 5165

MACMILLAN CANCER RELIEF
3 Angel Walk
London W6 9HX
Information line: 0845 601 6161
www.macmillan.org.uk

The free booklet "The Cancer Guide" gives useful contacts, phone numbers and other information.

MARIE CURIE CANCER CARE
28 Belgrave Square
London SW1X 8QG
Tel: 020 7235 3325
www.mariecurie.org.uk

WOMEN'S NATIONWIDE CANCER CONTROL CAMPAIGN
128 Curtain Road
London EC2
Information tape: 020 7729 4915
www.wnccc.org.uk

Index

Adriamycin: 55
Age: 6, 13, 14
Anaesthetic: 40, 46-47, 49
Anxiety—see Stress
Axillary lymph nodes: 38, 44, 51

Bloodstream: 11, 20, 21, 35
Bone marrow: 55, 56
Breast cancer,
    causes: 14-17
    diagnosis: 6-7, 22-23, 26-27, 37, 45
    frequency: 12-13
    in situ: 18, 76
    incidence: 12-13, 14-15
    invasive: 18-19, 44
    reactions to: 72-73, 74-75
    remission: 12, 69
    research: 22-23, 60
    support groups: 7, 43, 68, 70, 71, 78
    types of: 6, 18-21
Breastfeeding: 16
Breasts,
    cysts: 16, 19, 26, 29
    discharge: 26
    examination: 6, 27
    fibroadenomas: 16
    implants: 48-49
    lumps – see Breast tumours
    lymphatic system: 11, 21, 40, 43, 47, 52, 76
    nipple inversion: 26
    prostheses: 7, 66-67
    structure of: 10-11
    tumours: 10-11, 13, 16, 20-21, 26-27, 28, 34, 37, 40, 50, 77

Cancers: 12, 16, 17, 59
Cataracts: 59
Cells: 10, 14, 16, 18, 19, 21, 31, 35, 36, 51, 55, 56, 58
Children: 14-15, 72-73
Contraception: 16, 17
Counselling: 61, 68, 70
Cyclophosphamide, methotrexate and 5-fluorouracil (CMF): 55
Cystic carcinoma: 19
Cytotoxic drugs: 54

Depression: 7
Diet: 14, 46, 56, 57, 75
Distant spread: 34-35, 38, 50
Doctors: 18, 26, 36, 50, 68, 70, 75
Ductal carcinoma in situ (DCIS): 18

Exercise: 37, 64-65

Fertility: 56
Fitness—see Exercise

Genes: 10, 17, 22-23, 60, 61
Glands: 10
Goserelin: 61

Hair loss: 7, 53, 57, 66-67, 72
Heart disease: 60, 61
Holistic care: 36-37
Hormone replacement therapy (HRT): 17, 38, 59
Hormones: 17, 58-59
Hospices: 75
Hyperplasia: 16, 19, 76

Invasive ductal carcinoma: 19

Lobes: 10, 20
Lobular carcinoma in situ (LCIS): 18-19
Lobules—see Lobes
Local spread: 20-21, 38, 50, 68
Lymph nodes 11, 21, 35, 38, 41, 43, 44, 50
Lymphoedema: 45, 47, 53, 77

Medication,
    Herceptin: 60
    Tamoxifen: 58-59, 60-61
Menopause: 13, 17, 39, 50, 54, 55, 56, 58, 59, 61
Menstruation: 15, 50, 56
Metastases: 20-21, 38-39, 55, 77

Oestrogen: 15, 16-17, 50, 58
Oncogenes: 23
Oophorectomy: 60-61, 77
Operations—see Surgery
Osteoporosis: 17, 60
Ovarian ablation: 60

Index

Paget's disease: 19
Palliative care: 74-75, 77
Pneumonitis: 53
Pregnancy: 14-15, 44, 45
Progesterone: 16, 50, 58
Prophylaxis: 61
Psychologists: 36-37
Puberty: 26

Reconstructive surgery: 37, 43, 48-49, 69

Sentinel node mapping: 43, 44
Sexuality: 68-69
Smoking: 16
Specialists: 36-37
Stress: 7, 22, 57
Surgery: 37-49, 64, 67

Terminal illness: 74-75
Tests,
  biopsy: 30-31, 76
  fine needle aspiration cytology (FNAC): 30-31, 37
  magnetic resonance imaging (MRI): 29
  mammograms: 12-13, 14, 28-29, 36, 61, 77

ultrasound: 29, 30
Therapy,
  adjuvant: 38-39, 43, 45, 49, 50, 55, 58, 76
  chemotherapy: 6, 21, 36, 38, 39, 44, 50, 51, 52, 54-55, 56, 58, 69, 72, 76
  complementary therapy: 71
  hormone therapy: 6, 39, 44, 50, 51, 52, 54, 58-59
  neo-adjuvant: 51
  radiotherapy: 6, 20, 36, 38, 39, 40-41, 45, 50, 51, 52-53
Thrombosis: 59
Treatments,
  lumpectomy: 31, 38, 40-41, 44, 45, 51, 52, 68, 76
  massage: 71
  mastectomy: 38, 40-41, 42-43, 44, 49, 51, 61, 64, 67, 69, 77
  physiotherapy: 37, 64
  systemic treatment: 38-39, 43, 54-61, 77
  types of: 34-61

Weight: 56

Acknowledgements

Photographs: Amoena (UK) ltd 66; Marshall Editions/Iain Bagwell 26/27; Science Photo Library (Breast Screening Unit, Kings College Hospital, London) 31, (Colin Cuthbert) 57, (Cecil H Fox) 36/37, 45, 51, 73, (Simon Fraser) 46, (Dr. P. Marazzi) 41, (Larry Mulvehill) 52; N1H Custom Medical Stock Photo 34, 75, (Chris Priest) 24/25; (Quest) 7, 22, 39, 48, (Geoff Tompkinson) 28; gettyone Stone 17

Commissioned photography: Guglielmo Galvin

Edited and designed by Phoebus Editions, 72–80 Leather Lane, London EC1N 7TR

Thanks to Patsy North and Ros Newby for modelling for the photographs